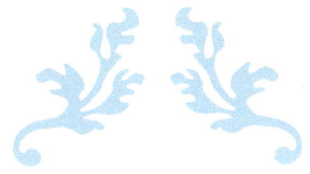

FIT @ 40

A guide to sustainable weight loss

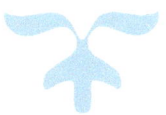

DAPO OJO

Contents

Preface

Introduction

To Self-improvement.

Preface

There are so many books out there that give numerous instructions on how to lose weight, stay fit and live a healthy life, however, they don't provide an engaging step-by-step guide, complete with real-life experience from the beginning of the journey to the point where you achieve your goals.

I began my weight loss / get fit journey at the age of 37 and arrived at the desired result just months before I turned 40, hence the title – Fit@40. It took this long because I was searching for answers, though it would have taken less time if I knew all what I know now. If you adopt this book as a guide to your personal weight loss journey, you would **achieve and sustain success** more efficiently.

Introduction

There are currently perhaps hundreds of millions of overweight, obese or morbidly obese people all over the world who are constantly seeking to change their bodies to a healthier, slimmer or toned version as they've often imagined themselves to be. Many have tried dieting, exercise, pills and even some extreme measures such as starving and wiring their teeth shut to completely prevent themselves from eating. These methods, which are often applied abruptly, without a doubt, lead to undesirable results or even expose the individuals to moderate or severe health risks such as Malnutrition, Dehydration, Constipation, Bone Loss, Fatigue, High Blood Pressure, amongst others – www.stylecraze.com (Sept. 19, 2017).

4

With the numerous weight loss plans available today, a great majority of these people still struggle to shed the excess weight permanently, simply because these plans have a negative rebounding effect once the individual deviates even slightly from it; *"more than 80 percent of people who have lost weight regain all of it, or more, after two years. Researchers at the University of California at Los Angeles analyzed 31 long-term diet studies and found that about two-thirds of dieters regained more weight within four or five years than they initially lost"* (Gretchen Voss, WOMEN'S HEALTH).

As it is, I'm yet to come across anyone who is willing or able to live on supplements in the form of snack bars, shakes and soups for the rest of their lives!

So, you may wonder what it is that I'm bringing on board that is new. The answer is simple – Nothing! What I intend to do is not to create a new "wow", but to share with you the **"how",** which has worked for me and others I have mentored, **to achieve and sustain your ideal body weight.**

My intention is to focus on the right lifestyle-modifying approach in a series of steps which are adaptable and easily sustainable, the challenges at each stage of progress and how you will be able to surmount them.

<u>Note:</u> I am not a trained medical practitioner and will not prescribe any treatment for any physiological or psychological condition with regards to weight management. I'm only about to share with you, my success story and how you can achieve yours.

Enjoy reading!

Chapter 1

Travails and Challenges

In the 80's, parts of the world hadn't taken to account the severity of the negative psychological effects of name-calling of an individual or a group of individuals with regards to what makes them "stand out", whether by their physical attributes, beliefs or origin *et cetera*, so there were no holds barred with the teasing. Standing at 4'9" and weighing about 55kg (121.25 lbs) at age 9, led to cat-calls like, "The big one", "Fat boy", "Fatty bum bum", "Mighty Igor" (famous sausage-eating IWA wrestler in the 80's) all had a negative impact on my self-confidence which led to shyness whilst in the midst of my peers. I remember often waiting to be alone in order to change clothes for PE (Physical Education) sessions and folding my arms across my chest to hide the bulges underneath while taking team photographs. This didn't last beyond elementary school, however, I saw the humour in it in secondary school as I got older and more matured, so it stopped bothering me. I guess I erroneously accepted it as 'just the way I am' believing that some people aren't just meant to be slim and fit and was lucky to quickly outgrow the negative feeling of being teased as not many people faced with a similar situation would have such fortitude. For some, it evolves to a level of stigma which they struggle with throughout their lives, however, the good thing is that they can do something about it and this book will provide the necessary information and support throughout the journey.

Notwithstanding the negative jibes from others, I had personal challenges too but it was more physical than emotional. My adolescent and teenage years, like it was and still is for most cultures worldwide, were a time of increased social activities with fashion playing an integral part. At some point, it was the "in thing" to wear very tight trousers and an oversized shirt. Needless to say, I had no problems with the shirts, however, it was an entirely different experience with the trousers. They would rip at the slightest exertive movement, mostly in the "sanctified" parts and cause me great embarrassment, so imagine my relief when "baggy" trousers became mainstream fashion!

Physical activity also was an area in which I couldn't perform optimally. My sport of choice was football (soccer) and though I had well above average skills for it, I was always outperformed by many of my less skillful peers who were slim, fit and agile. I remember being bumped to the second team as a result of this but it really wasn't such a big deal; it didn't take the fun out of the game thanks to my **positive mental attitude**. I knew deep down that I would be where I wanted to be on the team only if only I was slimmer and fitter and though I didn't yet know how to achieve this at that point, however, it helped me come to terms with the situation I was in, realizing that a change was necessary and in later life, the same positive mental attitude helped me lose weight and get fit.

A positive approach or mindset is a necessary ingredient to begin and sustain your weight loss / get fit journey. Challenges and obstacle will surely emerge at various stages of your journey but the good news is that they are not unsurmountable. With a **positive mental attitude** and complete **focus on your intended goal,** the end result will leave you looking and feeling healthier with a restored and immeasurable increase in self-confidence.

Life as an overweight individual

A great majority of people who fall in the overweight category often experience life in a way that people who fall within the "normal" weight range more often do not – they are super self-conscious. This self-consciousness always revs up when they find themselves in public. Even a completely innocent glance from a stranger stirs up negative thoughts that perhaps they're being checked out, assessed, disapproved of or even loathed. A continuous feeling of such indignation impacts negatively on self-confidence and may cause the individual to feel sub-standard and perhaps, recline into themselves and withdraw from public view to the privacy of their home where they do more damage to themselves by overindulging in emotional eating".

Jennifer Kromberg PsyD, a licensed Clinical Psychologist, in her write up on *Emotional Eating* in *Psychology Today* of September 18, 2013 indicated *Body Hate* as one of the factors responsible for this eating habit. She wrote, "*It may sound counterintuitive, but it's true: hating your body is one of the biggest factors in emotional eating. Negativity, shame and hatred rarely inspire people to make long-lasting great changes, especially when it comes to our bodies or our*

sense of self. Many people tell me they will stop hating

their body after *they reach their goal weight. I say you*

have to stop hating your body before *you can stop the*

emotional eating cycle". This scenario, however a

seemingly vicious cycle, is commonplace with millions

of people who find themselves in the overweight

category (*Binge eating is the most common eating*

disorder, affecting approximately two million

Americans, according to statistics from the National

Institute of Mental Health). They wish they could be

different but don't seem to be able to help themselves,

however, the truth of the matter is that they could be

different or better yet, effect a positive difference to

their physique and yes – they **can** do it.

Chapter Summary

- *You **can** achieve and sustain your ideal body weight.*
- *You need a **positive mental attitude** to succeed.*
- *It's a journey, **focus on your goal** and your self-confidence will be restored.*

Footnote: Your body is yours to love, by all means, love it!

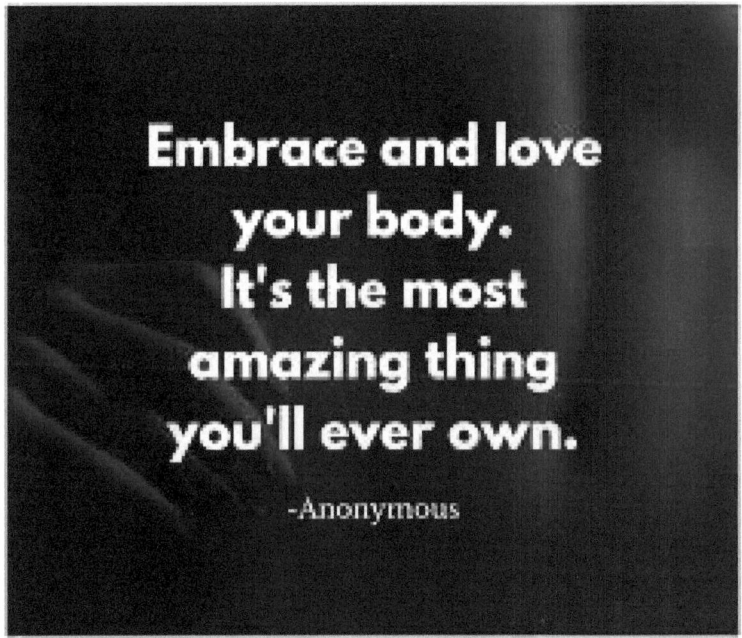

Photo source: www.wonderfabi.wordpress.com

Chapter 2

The Awakening

One morning, in February, 2013, I got on the scale and as it crunched the figures, I thought to myself, "this had better be good!" The figures finally registered at 116Kg (255.74lbs). Frankly speaking, this wouldn't be too bad if only I was seven feet tall, but standing at 5 feet 9.5 inches (1.75m), one thing was certain – I was obese! This experience turned out to be my wake-up call as it was the heaviest, I had ever been and at that point, I made up my mind to lose the excess weight and get fit.Now, registering at 113Kg (249.12lbs) in May, 2013, having lost 3Kg (6.61lbs) since February (perhaps from thinking about it all the time!), my goal

was to lose 30Kg (66.14lbs) in two years, that is 15Kg

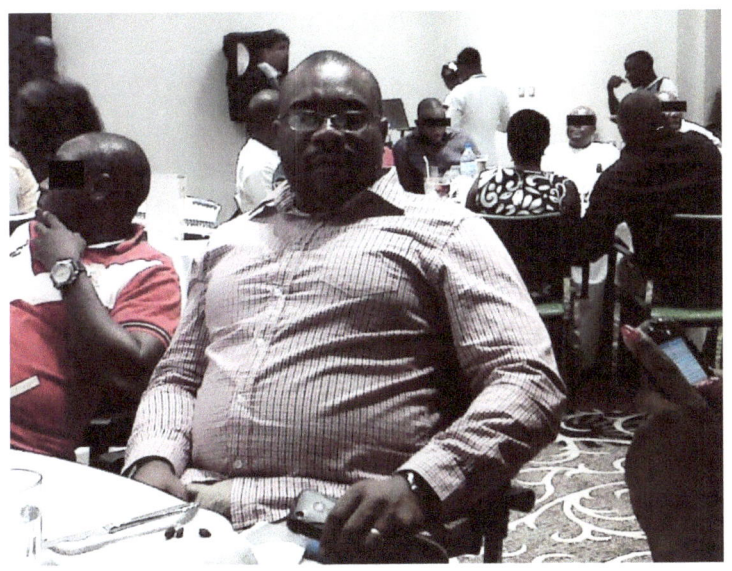

April, 2012.

(33.07lbs) in each year. Breaking it down further, that

is an average of 1.25Kg (2.76lbs) monthly over the

two-year period. Sounds easy, right? Of course, it's a

realistic plan!

You may wonder why I chose to lose 30Kg, well the reason is because I figured that pacing my progress in stages and accomplishing those stages within a specific time range would make the entire weight loss journey less burdensome. So, losing that much weight (30kg) would put me at 83Kg (183lbs), though 6Kg (13.23lbs) heavier than my ideal weight according to the Body Mass Index (BMI) calculation, however, I'd leave the category medically described as obese and further weight loss thereon, based on a new target, would be relatively less of a challenge.

Quick-fix Diet Plans

I had tried a couple of weight loss plans in the past and though I lost some weight whilst on the plan, but the moment I stopped, I would gain all the weight back plus extra. Talk about rebounding effect! So, what was I to do? I decided to approach the problem with an educated mind that is, to research into the human body as a way of understanding my own body, how it processes food and regulates weight. I came across some useful information in the course of my research and will elaborate on how I applied them in sequence as a fool proof template through the journey of actualizing my ideal weight.

Chapter summary

- *Set **realistic** and **achievable** weight loss goals.*
- *Give your weight loss goals **time** to foster – pace yourself.*
- *Quick-fix diet plans have no long-term benefits.*

Footnote: When you feel you've had enough, there's your wake-up call!

Photo source: www.bellaonthebeach.wordpress.com

Chapter 3

The Journey

Losing weight and getting fit is a journey that requires time to actualize the results of the effort put in. Striving to achieve your ideal weight isn't something that should be rushed, with the expectation of seeing results in a less than reasonable time frame. Bad eating habits and a sedentary lifestyle are two factors that contribute to being overweight and just as it actually takes time for the excess weight to pile on, so, on the flip side, there's no magic formula to undo the damage overnight – time is required.

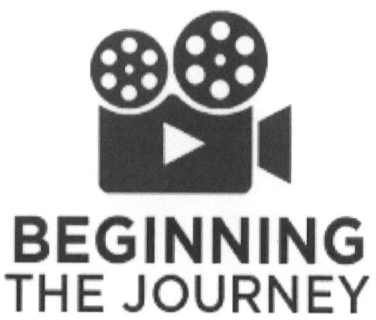

BEGINNING
THE JOURNEY

Photo source: www.ourterranova.com

Goals

Having done extensive research, I came to the

realization that in order to achieve my desired weight

and fitness, I had to modify my lifestyle in a series of

steps. The first step in my weight loss / get fit journey

was to set realistic goals, that is to say, a slow and

steady reduction in weight as the only sustainable way

to arrive at and permanently maintain the ideal body
weight, not to mention the most affordable too!

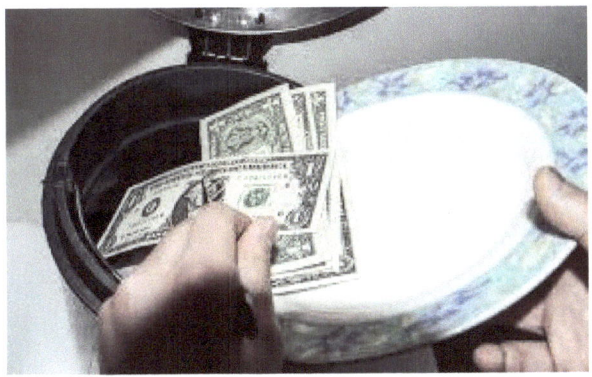

Photo source: www.newfoodmagazine.com

For the purpose of this book, I shall categorize
everyone who falls anywhere in the region of slightly
overweight to obese, simply as overweight.

In describing the distribution of excess weight in people
who are overweight, I would like to start with the
women – ladies first! With women, the excess weight

or fat is mostly deposited in the hips, thighs, buttocks, upper arms and the abdominal area while in men, it is mostly found in the chest, back and abdominal area. So, men and women who are overweight both have one thing in common – an excessive deposit of fat in the abdominal area, causing a disproportionate distension of that area. This abdominal fat, though less pronounced in women, contributes a reasonable portion to the overall excess weight of the body, therefore, a reduction in the deposit in this area would translate to a reasonable achievement in the weight loss journey. Ideally, though it is almost impossible to isolate a particular part of the body in which one wishes to trim off excess fat by non-surgical means, however, abdominal fat is relatively easily shed by taking into account the time of day that dinner is eaten as

suggested by the *Body Clock Diet*.

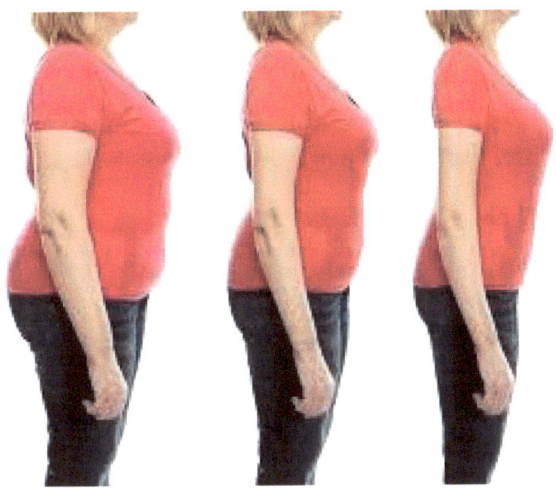

Photo source: www.glenmorehealthcare.com

Dinner is served!

If you are familiar with the Body Clock Diet, one of the

things it strongly propounds is an early dinner as this

gives the digestive system enough time to process the

food and allow the body to burn calories before bedtime, thereby having little or nothing to store as fat. With this in mind, **I decided to adopt a specific time for having dinner, believing that the earlier I had it before bedtime, the better off I'd be**. This proved to be correct. My strategy from the onset was to have a target and begin with what I could tolerate, then gradually work towards the set target as I became comfortable with the present condition. My target in this case was to have dinner no later than 5pm which was quite a challenge as I often ate just before bedtime at 11pm, so, I decided to start with 7pm and gradually work it back to 5pm. Dinner no later than 7pm isn't a stroll in the park for someone used to eating much later than that, but I had to start from somewhere, not forgetting the 5pm target and within days of sticking to my new dinner time, I noticed that my trousers became

looser in the waist, I slept more soundly and woke up

more refreshed and lighter on my feet – it was magical!

This experience provided me with the necessary boost

in confidence and determination to carry on with my

plan.

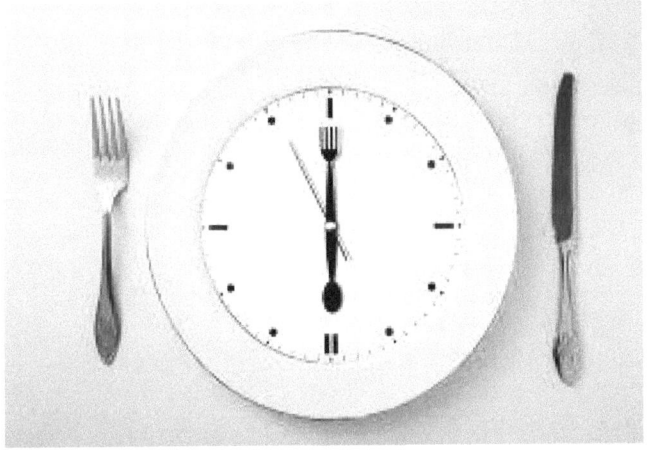

Photo source: www.sciencedaily.com

When I finally got used to eating dinner at 7pm, I

moved it down to 6:30pm and as a matter of fact, I

hardly noticed any difference in the time change and in

a matter of days, I moved it down to 6pm. Within the

next couple of weeks, I had moved it to 5:30pm and

then to 5pm. At this point, my mind started playing

tricks on me, perhaps because 5pm was my set target. I

would go to bed usually around 11pm with the feeling

that I needed to eat something to fall asleep. This was a

milestone that proved a bit of a challenge, it wasn't

easy but I fought it – and won!

It took months for me to get used to eating dinner at

5pm but my body eventually got used to the time

regime and gradually, my mind followed suit. I no

longer felt the need to have food in my stomach in

order to fall asleep, in fact, the reverse was the case as I

wouldn't be able to fall asleep unless my stomach was

completely empty, even to the point of being slightly hungry.

The gains (or losses in this case) of an early dinner were astounding! I lost 2 and a half inches off my waist and belly and within four months, I had lost 8Kg (17.64lbs). This may not sound like a lot of weight and inches to lose given the time it took, but when you consider that your body has "reprogramed" itself not to gain it back owing to your lifestyle modification, then you realize that it is quite an achievement.

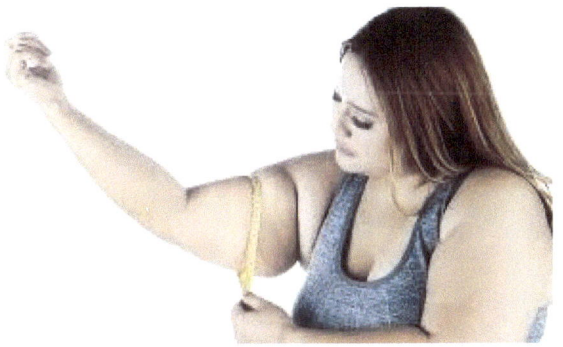

Photo source: www.pritikin.com

Hunter Gatherers

The term, "hunter gatherers" is used to describe our ancestors who lived hundreds of thousands of years ago, owing greatly to their lifestyles. As it was at that time of the early humans, just as it still is today, the most important aspect for survival was self-preservation with three basic necessities: food, clothing and shelter and in my opinion, food ranks foremost of all three. History teaches us that they subsisted on flesh from other animals and whatever they could scrounge in form of nuts, seeds and various parts of plants which they discovered to be edible. Scientific theories have emerged based on the studies of these early humans to help us understand their lifestyles and nutrition leading to such findings as that which is attributed to Peter D'adamo, a Naturopathic Doctor and author of the book – *Eat Right for Your Type*. He suggested that we need to consider our blood group in selecting different food types that prove most beneficial to us. I found his theory quite interesting and believed it could work, so I decided to apply it on my journey.

Like the great majority of people in the world, I am a blood type O and Dr. D'adamo theorized that individuals in this category require a lot of proteins in their diet, especially animal proteins in form of lean meats and other protein sources such as lentils including various bean types, complemented with vegetablcs and fruits, while also limiting foods made from wheat and grains. This coincides with information I got from several health write-ups I came across, stating the benefits of a protein-based breakfast as it sets the tone, so to speak, for the body's metabolism and calorie burn throughout the day. Also, an early protein-based dinner (5:00 pm in my case) proved beneficial as it leaves enough time to further burn calories before bedtime and also taking advantage of nature's gift to us humans in the sense that the body is hardly able to store proteins, rather, any excess of it is metabolized and excreted. Now, that leaves us with the issue of lunch. As energy levels begin to dip around mid-day, a carbohydrate-based meal proved to provide the necessary boost in energy required to sustain daily activity. Thinking percentages, what worked for me was approximately 40% complex carbs, 30% protein and 30% fruits and vegetables with as much water throughout the day as I could tolerate. This strategy, however, worked for someone I mentored who happens to be a blood type B, hence, my observation and as dieticians often propound, is that a healthy eating plan

consisting wholly of a balanced diet generally works

for anyone, though certain foods and food groups,

based on research conducted by the good doctor, really

may be more beneficial, otherwise, retrogressive to

particular blood types regarding healthy weight

sustenance.

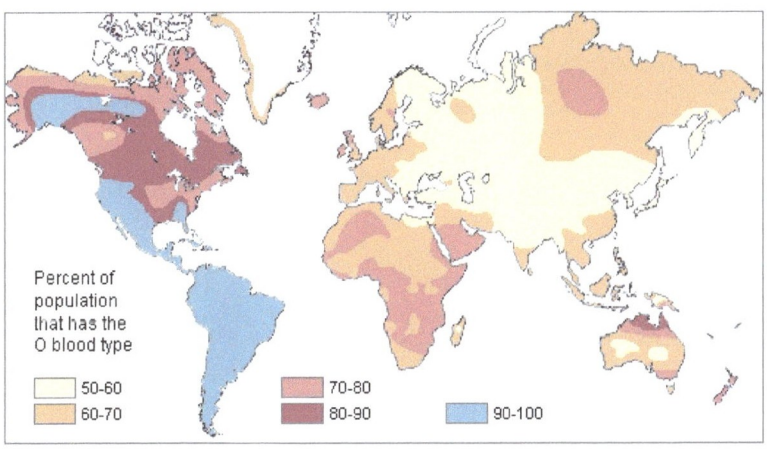

Image source: www2.palomar.edu

Cutting back

As mentioned earlier, I was able to achieve further weight loss not only wholly based on timing and the food types I chose to eat, but what also proved to be an active catalyst to the weight loss process was the quantity of food at every meal. To illustrate, take two individuals for instance, "A" and "B". Let's assume that both are the same age, gender, blood type, race, height, consume approximately the same number of calories and perform the same level of daily physical activity, however, "A" could fall within the limits of normal weight on the BMI scale while "B" could be overweight. "A" could perhaps consume even more calories and perform less daily physical activity than "B" and still wouldn't be overweight. Obviously, something else is at play – metabolism and energy expenditure owing to personal body chemistry. To be in the same weight category as "A", "B" would have to, more importantly, consume less calories, otherwise perform more physical daily activities. This example is a scenario I had seen personally because even though I wasn't really a big eater as far as big eating goes, I was overweight, actually obese and a few people I knew, who ate a whole lot more, were practically half my size. Basically, you need to gradually understand your own body with regards to **food types and quantity, energy expenditure** due to your **level of physical activity** and also your **metabolic rate** as you progress on the weight loss journey.

It is important to note that all strategies in the weight loss journey are best applied in a gradual manner so as to allow the body acclimatize to the change. Just as in

the case of bringing forward my dinner time from

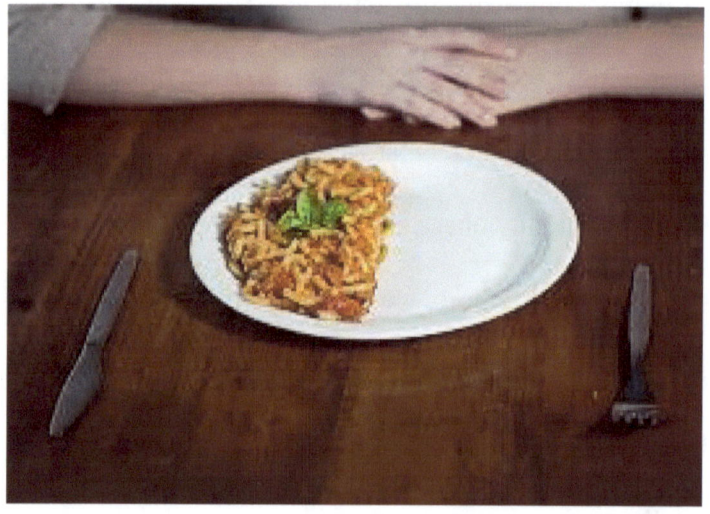

Photo source: www.istockphoto.com

7:00pm to 5:00pm, so it was with the reduction of food

quantity – gradually. When I had established and gotten

comfortable with my meal-type option, I proceeded to

reduce the quantity eaten at a time. I began with a 25% reduction, that is, I would divide my meal into four parts and eat three parts of it, leaving out one part. Once again, I didn't experience any challenge in such a subtle change and in a couple of weeks, I applied a 30% then progressed to a 40% reduction a few weeks thereafter, which I maintained for a few months. During this period, I continued to lose weight consistently albeit slowly as the size and volume of my stomach also shrunk.

A couple of months down the line, I noticed that I wasn't losing any more weight, I had hit a plateau on my weight loss journey so I needed to do something different to get back on track.

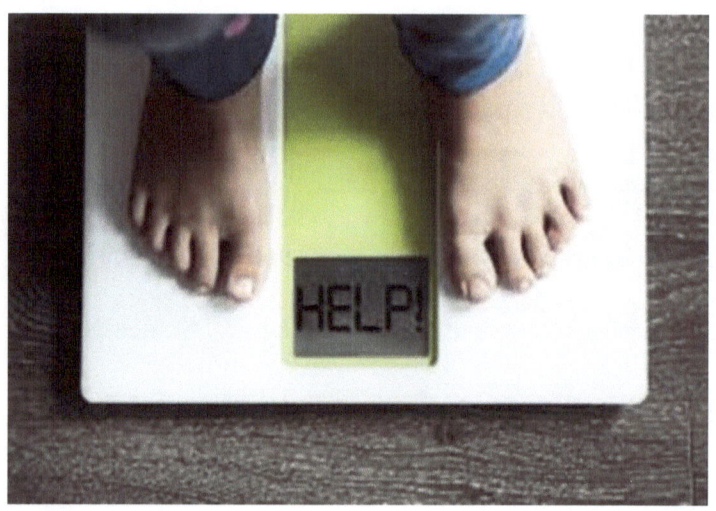

Photo source: www.forbes.com

More is less

This may sound strange, but what I proceeded to do was to change from eating three times daily to five times! Yes, I began eating five times daily but it all summed up to less food than when I ate three times. Bear in mind that before I made the decision to increase the frequency of meals, I was only consuming 60% of what I initially considered as a normal sized meal. So, what I did was to cut my breakfast in half and either have the other half for lunch or eat half of my lunch at the time of day. The same thing applied to dinner as well but nothing afterwards. In between these meals, I would have a healthy snack of about 100 – 120 calories to keep the hunger pangs at bay and drink as much water as I could tolerate throughout the day. This entire strategy of five daily meals summed up to be less food than when I ate three times and I got accustomed to it relatively quicker than the prior changes of food quantity and dinner time. The result was astonishing! I was quickly propelled off the plateau and my weight just kept on dropping. I didn't do anything else in a way of altering my eating habit because I had finally arrived at a solution that worked. I kept at it and weighed myself exactly one year from the time I commenced on the weight loss journey and was ecstatic to discover that I had lost exactly 15kg (33.07lbs). Again, one may erroneously judge that 15kg isn't a great deal of weight to lose in an entire year, but when you consider the fact that you won't gain it back owing to your modified relationship with food and your body's response to processing it, in addition to a super revved up metabolism, it indicates a huge success.

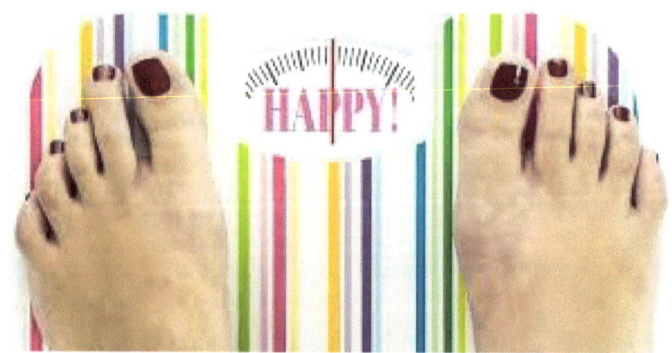

Photo source: www.weightlossresources.co.uk

Having adopted this as an eating lifestyle, my body just does the rest by burning stored fat to provide me with energy to sustain my daily activities. I will elaborate more on my activities in the following chapter, however, it is pertinent to mention that I lost another 15kg (33.07lbs) the following year and 8kg (17.64lbs) six months thereafter. I currently weigh 78kg (171.96lbs) which is just 1.7kg (3.7lbs) more than what is required for my BMI to be exactly 24.9, considered medically within the ideal or normal range.

I'd like to believe that my muscle density has a part to play in the 1.7kg (3.7lbs) in question owing to activities I perform regularly (next chapter), otherwise, I'll just accept the 97.8% success...for now!

Chapter Summary

- *Achieving steady weight loss takes time – pace yourself.*
- *Eat dinner as early in the day as possible.*
- *Certain food types may prove beneficial to certain blood groups* (Dr. Peter D'damo).
- *Try and understand your own body and what it needs.*
  Begin with what you can tolerate and make improvements gradually.

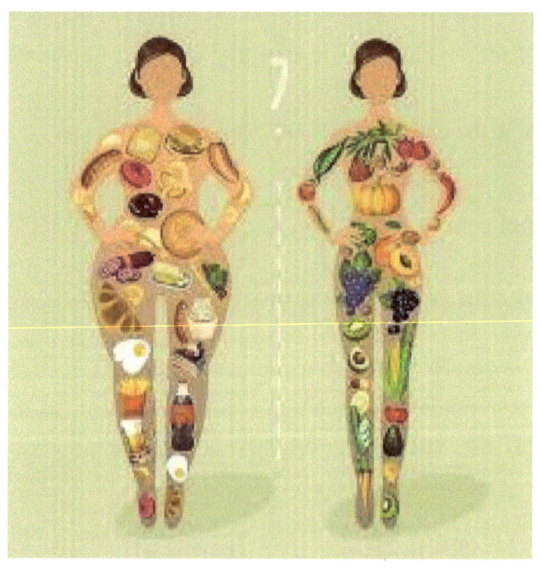

Photo source: www.drpia.com

Chapter 4

Exercise

Yeah, good ol' fashioned exercise!

I know that many people, whether in the overweight category or not, would shriek at the mere mention of the word, "exercise" but think about it; our early ancestors were toned and fit, not only because they ate just enough to essentially sustain their lives, but also because they did a lot of hunting. Bear in mind that they didn't have high powered rifles with sniper scopes and they hadn't invented bows and arrows or traps, meaning that they had to chase down their prey over considerably great distances and finally put it down.

Imagine chasing a deer long and far enough to subdue

it, then having to carry it back over that same distance,

to the homestead or cave to be prepared as a meal.

Now, if that isn't exercise, then I'm not sure what

qualifies!

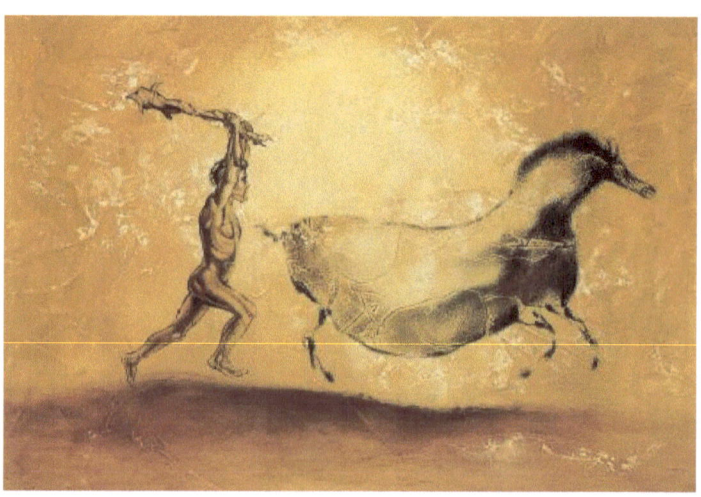

Photo source: www.strengthsensei.com

I will not cease to propound that everything applicable in this weight loss journey, ought to be done gradually with periodic increase in intensity as tolerated. Having said that, you don't need to begin exercising like an Olympics bound athlete, rather, a break away from perhaps daily sedentary routine by introducing a tolerable physical activity would suffice. I have realized that the secret to efficient exercise is to do what you enjoy doing so it doesn't appear to be a burden. In my case, I've always done a form of exercise fairly frequently – I play Squash three times a week, a routine which began long before I decided to actively begin the process to lose weight. It just happens to be a physical activity I so much enjoy and is part of my lifestyle, so to speak.

As at the time I decided to begin my weight loss

journey, I had been playing squash passively for over

28 years, however, I was still overweight, reason being

what we discussed in the previous chapter – food

quantity, type and dinner time. Apparently, I was

consuming more calories than what was required

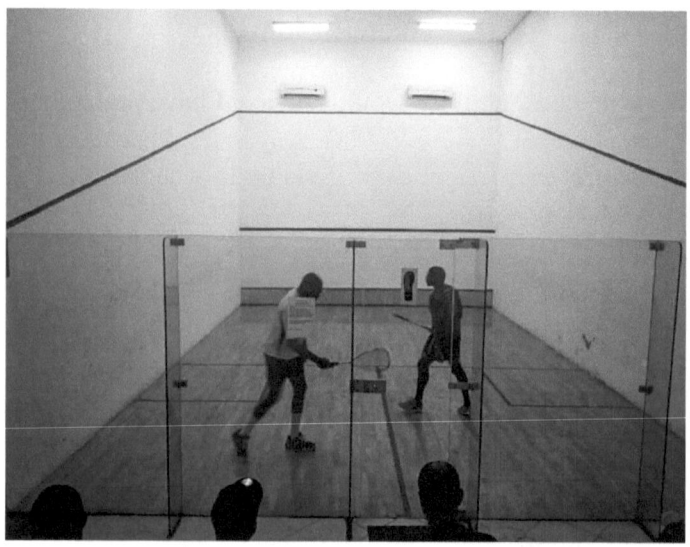

to keep my weight within healthy limits even though I

was physically active. This is not an attempt to

underscore the benefits of exercise, but just to emphasize that even with exercise, one still needs to have healthy eating habits which in my opinion, caters for perhaps 80% of healthy weight regulation, so as to further enhance the efficacy of exercise. I probably would have been much more overweight if I hadn't done any form of exercise at all.

Dr. Anthony Balduzzi, author of *The Fit father Project*, highlights nutrition as the most important factor in weight loss and management for men over the age of 40, as illustrated in his diagram (The Fat Loss Pyramid), with Daily Activity and Formal Exercise following closely.

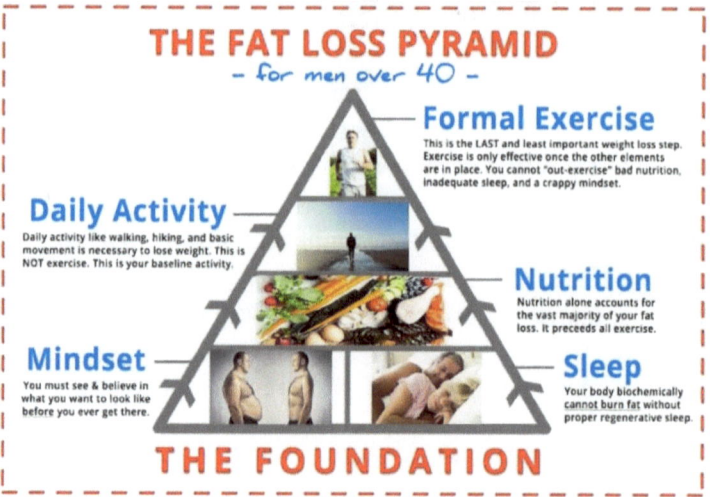

Photo source: www.fitfatherproject.com

Intensify

Following my decision to lose excess weight, I gradually increased the intensity and duration of playing squash. Playing time usually, was 30 minutes three times a week and as I continued to lose weight and get fit, it gradually increased to an hour on

Mondays and Wednesdays followed by 15 lengths of freestyle swimming in a 33-meter (109 ft.) pool and an hour thirty minutes of squash on Fridays followed by 30 minutes in the sauna. I've added a routine to my exercise for about a month now, which is, five days a week of 100 push-ups, 100 reverse triceps push-ups and 500 sit-ups. Once again, I didn't begin at that level, I started with what I could tolerate and gradually built up on it.

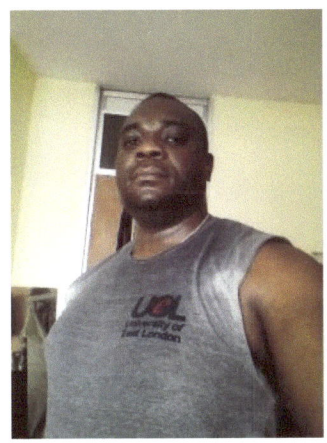 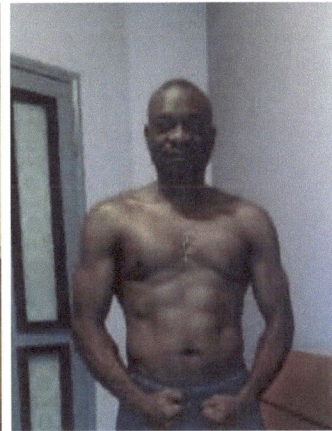

May, 2013.   *August, 2015.*

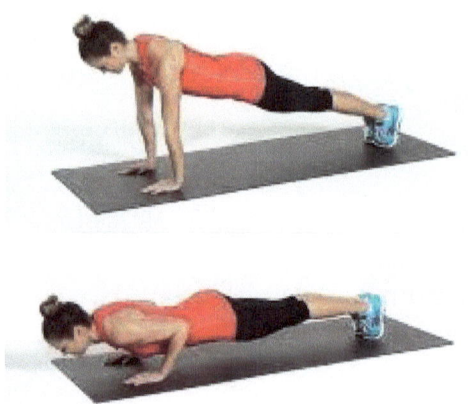

Push up – Photo source: www.popsugar.com

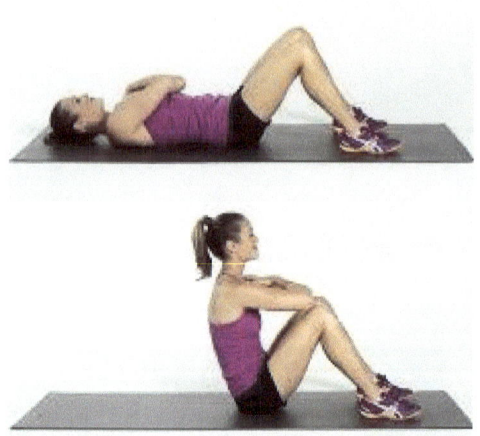

Sit up – Photo source: www.popsugar.com

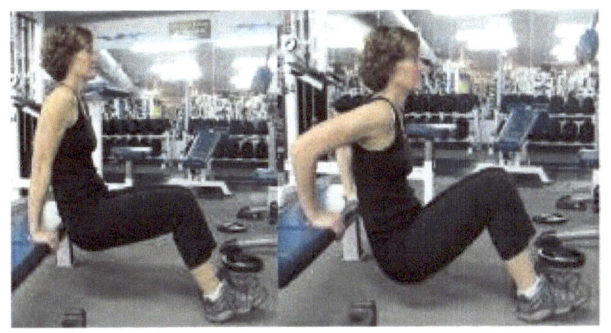

Reverse triceps push up – Photo source:

www.burnthefatinnercircle.com

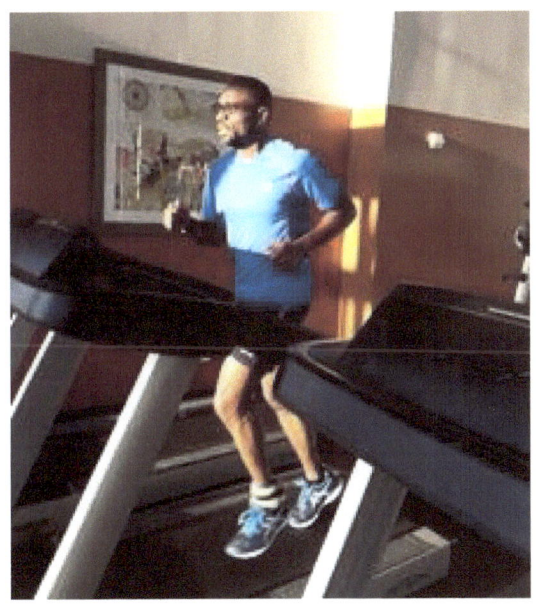

December, 2018.

Please bear in mind that whether you're new to exercise or not, as long as you're overweight, you should commence with a form of exercise that is low-impact, preventing any direct consequences to your joints, especially the knees. So, instead of running or skipping, you may consider a brisk walk (with or without the dog) or swimming, low-impact aerobics, dance aerobics or simply any activity that requires increased physical effort, just as long as you get to break sweat.

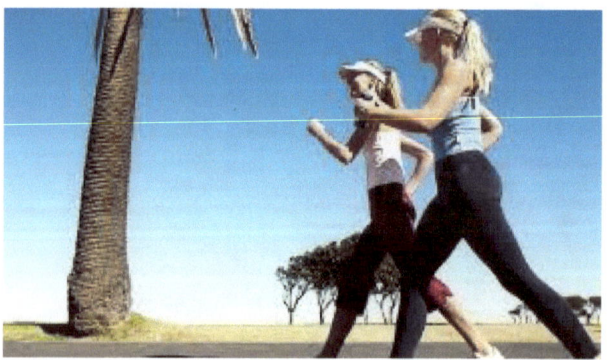

Photo source: www.health.com

However, I strongly suggest that you **consult your physician before embarking on any form of exercise** so as to rule out risks of any underlying medical condition(s).

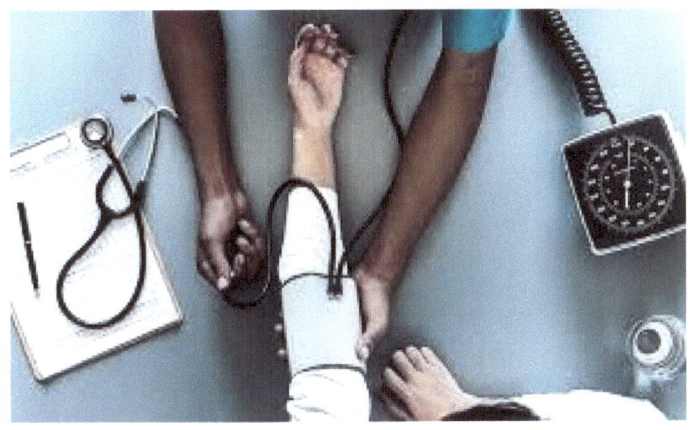

Photo source: www.abbeyskitchen.com

Chapter summary

- *Exercise ought not be tasking – enjoy it.*
- *Begin with low-impact cardio then gradually intensify as tolerated.*

- *Adopt different forms of exercise.*
- *Be consistent.*

Footnote: Take care of your body, its your only

permanent home!

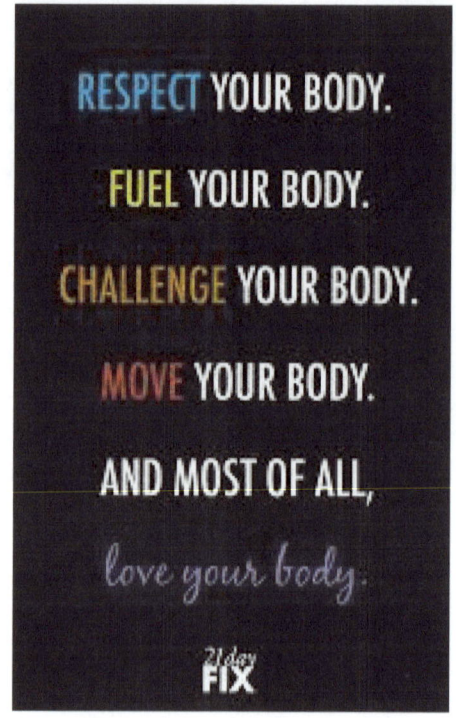

Photo source: www.pinterest.com

Chapter 5

Determination

You've just read the summary of my weight loss journey in a nutshell, which hopefully, has provided you with enough encouragement to embark on your own personal journey. I emphasize on the word, "personal" because the decision to lose weight and get fit is a personal one in which you need to make up your own mind, by yourself, rather than being coerced into it by negative comments and side glances or outright stares from other people, or the need to adopt a quick fix approach so as to be able to fit into a dress or a pair of pants for an occasion you want to attend in a week or two. These negative scenarios in turn, cause you to project a negative image

of yourself which could lead to emotional struggles and make weight loss too much of a challenge. Take charge of yourself, you are in control!

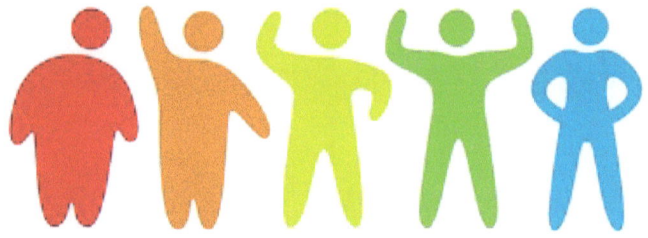

Photo source: www.nutritionrx.ca

Power to change

We are all at different points in the journey through life but with the same certainty - we cannot change our past. From the moment we were born, right up to this very moment, there is absolutely nothing we can alter, it is all out of our control, however, from this point on and right up to the very end, when we exit this world, we are in control of almost everything – with a few exceptions, of course. For instance, we cannot change our physical attributes of height or race as these are genetically encoded in our DNA, but we have the total and absolute control in changing and regulating our weight.

Once you believe that you can achieve this and you're willing to put in the required effort with a positive mindset, believe me, you've already covered a great distance in the weight loss journey.

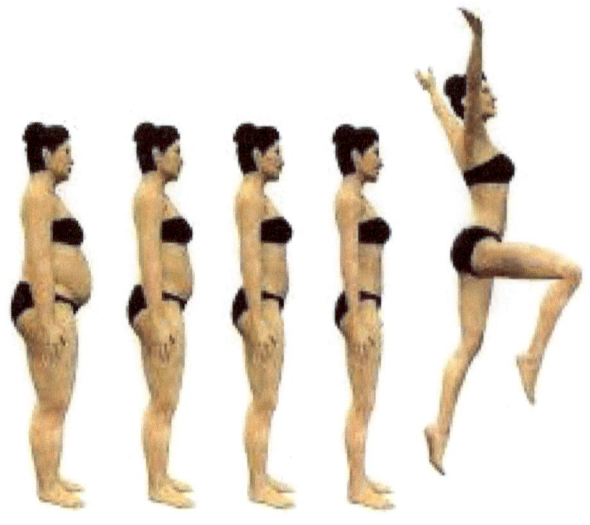

Photo source: www.therootdoctor.se

Let's get started!

As I mentioned earlier, the aim of this book is to inform

you **how I was able to achieve weight loss and**

prevent myself from further weight gain. I could stop

right here but wouldn't feel that I've done a complete

job, so I'd like you to experience a less cumbersome

weight loss journey by providing more information in greater detail.

The "wonder" App

Just before I embarked on my weight loss journey, I had a conversation with my sister, Mo, who was losing weight and getting fit herself. She went from a dress size 16 to a size 0 in just over two years! She introduced me to an app, *My Fitness Pal* (myfitnesspal) and swore by everything holy that it would prove beneficial. *"How the heck am I gonna lose weight with an app!"*, I wondered aloud, but she was persistent, so I installed it on my tablet and gave it a shot – it was remarkable! It requires the user to enter details of gender, age, height, weight, lifestyle (sedentary, active, *et cetera*) and target weight. It then calculated the amount of calories, percentage of proteins, carbohydrates and fats and also water to be consumed daily to reach the ideal weight over a prescribed period of time. This may sound complicated but it is as easy as breathing! It requires you to log in whatever you've eaten for breakfast, lunch, dinner or snack time and it tells you how many calories and food types it contains, the amount you have left to consume for the day or if you've gone overboard, as the case may be. If you do exercise, it tells you how many calories you've burned based on the type and duration of such exercise. Believe me, this app proved to be a practical guide to a systematic reduction of excess calorie intake and paved the way to the commencement of my weight loss journey, just as it would for you too!

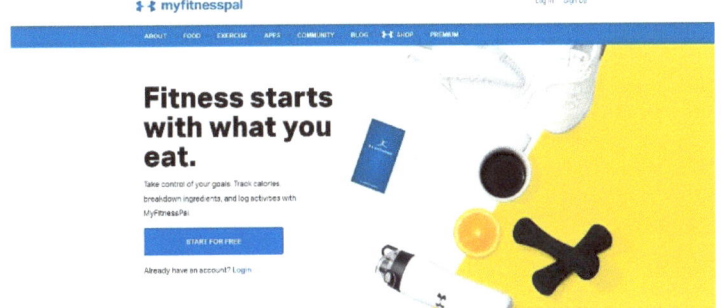

Photo source: www.myfitnesspal.com

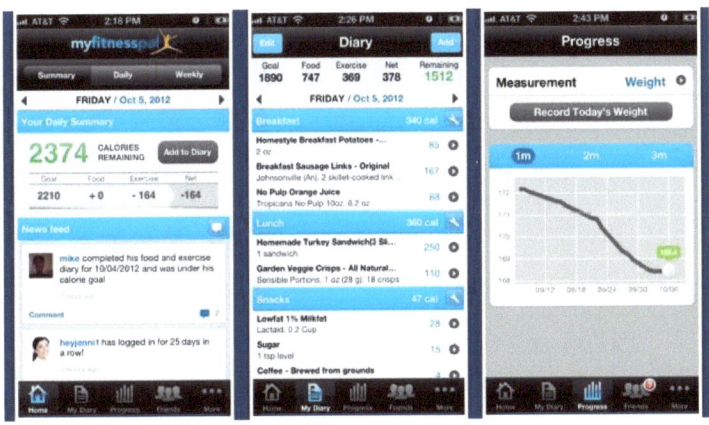

Photo source: www.getthegloss.com

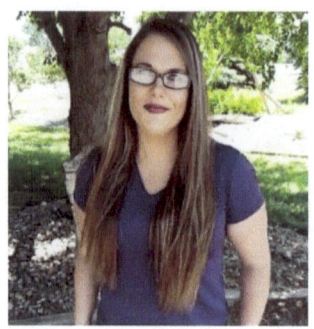

Education helped her lose 30 pounds

MyFitnessPal gave me a wake up call to the way I was eating and made things clear what I needed to change.

-Stephanie

Photo source: www.myfitnesspal.com

Chapter summary

- *Your weight loss / get fit journey is a personal decision – its all about you;*
- *You can change your body – the power is in you;*
- *Keep track of your calorie intake and physical activity;*
- *You will succeed!*

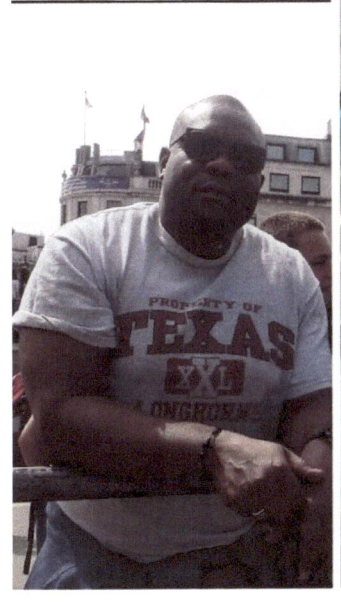
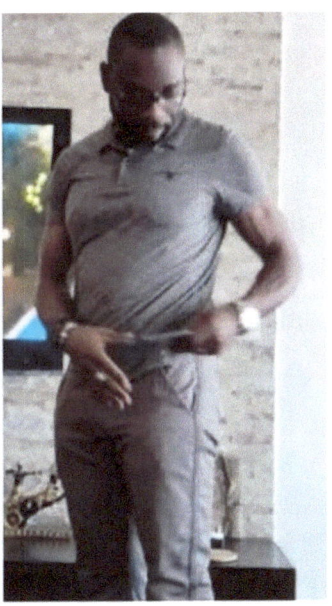

August, 2013.   *November, 2018.*

Chapter 6

Staying focused

You will experience challenges and periods of low enthusiasm on you journey but it is most important to **stay focused on the goal**. One of the challenges I experienced personally was hitting a plateau at various stages especially when I got comfortable with the eating condition at that time. Whenever I found myself in such a situation, I would introduce another rule just as I mentioned in Chapter 3 – I would do something like reduce the quantity of food at every meal, reduce the quantity of carbohydrates and fill up with more protein and vegetables or I would just bring forward my dinner time. What is important is that you focus on your desired result and as much as possible, enjoy the journey with the assurance that success is certain.

You may celebrate milestones as this reinforces your sense of accomplishment and thereafter, move on to the next challenge – one you can tolerate then gradually increase in intensity until you arrive at your goal.

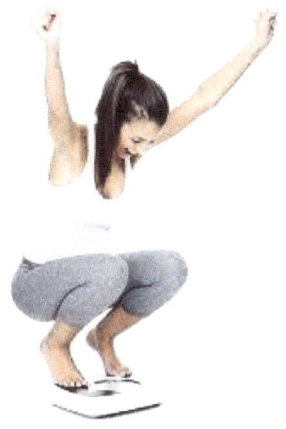

Photo source: www.genesishealthsolutions.net

Lifestyle maintenance

When you finally arrive at your goal, at that very point, eating habits with regards to food types, quantity and mealtimes coupled with your level of physical activity, altogether become your lifestyle which you must maintain in order to sustain the results. This, however, is the least challenging part of the entire journey because you would be so pleased with the results of your accomplishment and your body would have acclimatized to the great changes in a series of small steps that you've made over time and deviating even slightly from your eating regimen may not come easy. That is to say, even if you desire to put on some weight, it may not come easily without an appreciable level of effort. That's good news! I experienced this myself at a time after I had achieved my desired result. I brought my dinner time to 2:00pm and lost 4kg (8.8lbs) in a

couple of weeks. Needless to say, I felt underweight at

74kg (163lbs) as my bone structure became visible. I'd

find myself swaying and struggling to maintain balance

when outside on a windy day. It wasn't until when my

ribs became prominent that I decided to put on some

weight. I tried to eat more at mealtimes but my stomach

had already shrunk to a point where it could only

accommodate relatively small amounts of food. Binge

eating was extremely difficult for the same reasons.

Also, I tried eating later than usual but that too proved

impossible as I was already used to eating at certain

times during the day and my stomach would "lock"

itself at 4:00pm. I then resorted to eating high calorie

foods with no exercise whatsoever and managed to gain

back 3kg (6.6lbs) over a two-month period!

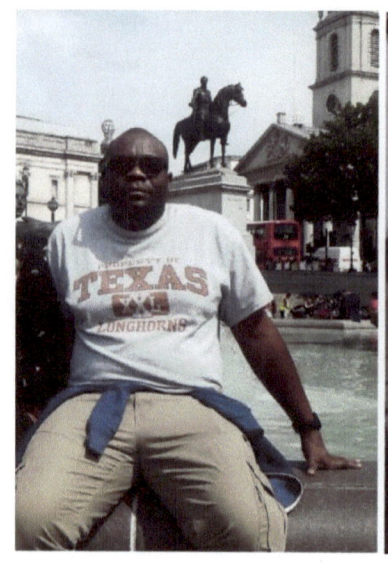 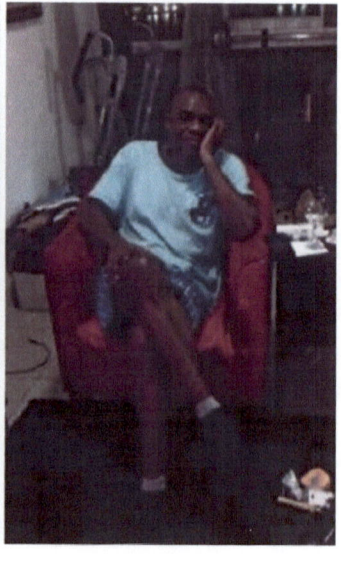

August, 2013.   *July, 2015.*

Conclusion

I hope this small book (with a big solution!) provides you with enough information based on my personal experience and those I've mentored, to proceed on your personal weight loss / get fit journey. I'd like to summarize it by providing you with a template of food reduction applicable over a six-month period as a way of kick-starting your journey. Once again, the strategy is to gradually decrease the quantity of food to what you can tolerate and when you feel comfortable with it over a few weeks, you could proceed to make further reductions. Continue this process repeatedly until you finally arrive at the quantity of food that works for you as will be indicated by your desired weight goal.

Meal size	Duration (minimum)	
¾ of present consumption	21 days – 1 month	
2/3 of present consumption	6 - 8 weeks	
½ of present consumption	6 – 8 weeks	
1/3 of present consumption	1 month and beyond as Maintenance	

Photo source: www.researchgate.net

(food dishes for illustration purposes only).

Kindly note that you may stop at any milestone of food reduction when you reach your goal weight and maintain it there and not necessarily go all the way to 1/3 of your present consumption.

So, ladies and gentlemen, that's all I did to lose weight and get **Fit @ 40**…and its not rocket science!

Have a safe and pleasant journey!

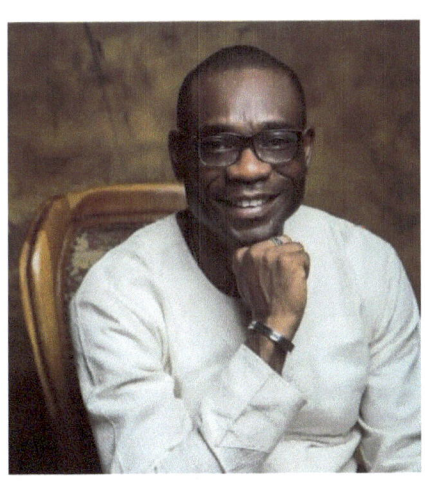

40rty.Fit@gmail.com